Acid Reflux Diet

An Absolute Beginner's 5-Step Plan, With a Foods List, Sample Recipes, and a 7-Day Meal Plan

copyright © 2023 Tyler Spellmann

All rights reserved No part of this book may be reproduced, or stored in a retrieval system, or transmitted in any form or by any means, electronic, mechanical, photocopying, recording, or otherwise, without express written permission of the publisher.

Disclaimer

By reading this disclaimer, you are accepting the terms of the disclaimer in full. If you disagree with this disclaimer, please do not read the guide.

All of the content within this guide is provided for informational and educational purposes only, and should not be accepted as independent medical or other professional advice. The author is not a doctor, physician, nurse, mental health provider, or registered nutritionist/dietician. Therefore, using and reading this guide does not establish any form of a physician-patient relationship.

Always consult with a physician or another qualified health provider with any issues or questions you might have regarding any sort of medical condition. Do not ever disregard any qualified professional medical advice or delay seeking that advice because of anything you have read in this guide. The information in this guide is not intended to be any sort of medical advice and should not be used in lieu of any medical advice by a licensed and qualified medical professional.

The information in this guide has been compiled from a variety of known sources. However, the author cannot attest to or guarantee the accuracy of each source and thus should not be held liable for any errors or omissions.

You acknowledge that the publisher of this guide will not be held liable for any loss or damage of any kind incurred as a result of this guide or the reliance on any information provided within this guide. You acknowledge and agree that you assume all risk and responsibility for any action you undertake in response to the information in this guide.

Using this guide does not guarantee any particular result (e.g., weight loss or a cure). By reading this guide, you acknowledge that there are no guarantees to any specific outcome or results you can expect.

All product names, diet plans, or names used in this guide are for identification purposes only and are the property of their respective owners. The use of these names does not imply endorsement. All other trademarks cited herein are the property of their respective owners.

Where applicable, this guide is not intended to be a substitute for the original work of this diet plan and is, at most, a supplement to the original work for this diet plan and never a direct substitute. This guide is a personal expression of the facts of that diet plan.

Where applicable, persons shown in the cover images are stock photography models and the publisher has obtained the rights to use the images through license agreements with third-party stock image companies.

Table of Contents

Introduction	7
What Is Acid Reflux?	10
Difference Between GERD and Acid Reflux	10
Causes of Acid Reflux	11
Symptoms of Acid Reflux	12
Medical Treatments for Acid Reflux	14
Natural Remedies for Acid Reflux	15
Lifestyle Changes to Manage Acid Reflux	16
What Is the Acid Reflux Diet?	18
Principle of Acid Reflux Diet	18
Benefits of the Acid Reflux Diet	21
Disadvantages of the Acid Reflux Diet	27
How to Get Started with the Acid Reflux Diet	30
Step 1: Understand Your Condition	30
Step 2: Identify Trigger Foods	32
Step 3: Design Your Diet	33
Step 4: Stay Hydrated	35
Step 5: Monitor Your Progress	36
Foods to Eat	38
Foods to Avoid	39
Sample Meal Plan	41
Sample Recipes	44
Banana Oatmeal	45
Grilled Chicken Salad	46
Baked Salmon with Broccoli and Quinoa	48
Scrambled Egg Whites on Toast	49
Turkey and Spinach Wrap	50
Grilled Fish with Sweet Potatoes	51
Spinach Pineapple Smoothie	53

Quinoa Salad	54
Roasted Chicken with Carrots and Rice	55
Whole Grain Cereal with Almond Milk	57
Tuna Salad	57
Baked Cod with Asparagus	59
Greek Yogurt with Honey and Almonds	60
Chicken Vegetable Soup	61
Grilled Shrimp Skewers	63
Teriyaki Shrimp Sushi Bowl	64
Chicken and Mushroom Cheese Bake	66
Maple BBQ Salmon	68
Caribbean Fish Tacos	70
Icy Mango Smoothie	72
Conclusion	**74**
FAQs	**77**
References and Helpful Links	**79**

Introduction

Are you frequently tormented by a burning sensation in your chest that makes enjoying meals a challenging task? Do you often find yourself waking up in the middle of the night, clutching your chest, with a sour taste in your mouth? If these symptoms strike a chord, you may be one of the millions dealing with a common yet unsettling condition known as acid reflux.

Acid reflux or GERD (Gastroesophageal reflux disease) is a prevalent health issue affecting people globally. While over-the-counter medications and antacids provide momentary relief, they don't address the root cause. But, what if the key to managing acid reflux lies not in your medicine cabinet but on your dining table? Yes, the solution could be as simple as tweaking your diet. By understanding the dietary triggers and incorporating acid reflux-friendly foods, one can significantly manage, if not entirely prevent, the occurrence of acid reflux.

Imagine savoring your favorite meals without the constant fear of triggering another bout of heartburn. Envision nights where sleep comes easy without the discomfort of acid creeping up your throat. It's not just a dream but a potential reality for those suffering from acid reflux. With an appropriate acid reflux diet, it's possible to regain control over your digestive health and live a life unhampered by the fear of heartburn.

In this guide, we will talk about the following:

- What is Acid Reflux?
- Causes and symptoms of Acid Reflux
- Medical treatments and natural remedies for Acid Reflux
- Lifestyle changes to manage Acid Reflux
- What is an Acid Reflux Diet?
- Principles of Acid Reflux Diet
- Benefits and disadvantages of Acid Reflux Diet
- Foods to eat and to avoid
- Sample meal plan and recipes

So, are you ready to dive deep into the world of acid reflux and understand how simple dietary changes can turn around your life? This comprehensive guide aims to guide you through the science behind acid reflux, the role of diet in managing it, and how to make informed food choices that keep heartburn at bay.

Together, let's embark on this journey towards better digestive health. Let's explore the world of acid reflux, understand its triggers, and discover the power of diet in controlling it. Your first step towards a life free from the constraints of heartburn starts here. Keep reading to find out more about acid reflux and how you can manage it through diet and natural remedies.

What Is Acid Reflux?

Acid reflux, medically known as gastroesophageal reflux disease (GERD), is a prevalent digestive disorder where stomach acid or bile irritates the food pipe lining. This condition occurs when the lower esophageal sphincter, a ring of muscle that acts as a valve between the esophagus and stomach, doesn't close properly.

This allows harmful stomach acid to back up into the esophagus, causing a burning sensation commonly known as heartburn. If ignored, acid reflux can lead to serious health complications, including damage to the esophagus. However, with proper understanding and lifestyle modifications, individuals can effectively manage this condition.

Difference Between GERD and Acid Reflux

Acid reflux and GERD (Gastroesophageal Reflux Disease) are often used interchangeably, but they are not the same.

Acid reflux is a common occurrence where stomach acid or bile flows back into the food pipe, causing a burning sensation known as heartburn. This can happen to anyone occasionally, especially after consuming certain types of food or drink.

GERD, on the other hand, is a chronic, more severe form of acid reflux. It's diagnosed when acid reflux occurs more than twice a week and results in inflammation in the esophagus. GERD can lead to more serious complications like esophageal ulcers or a condition called Barrett's esophagus, which increases the risk of esophageal cancer.

In essence, all people with GERD have acid reflux, but not everyone with acid reflux has GERD. The frequency and severity of symptoms are key factors in diagnosing GERD.

Causes of Acid Reflux

Understanding the causes of acid reflux is essential in managing its symptoms and potential complications. Here are several known factors that can trigger acid reflux:

- **Frequent acid reflux:** This is the primary cause of GERD. When stomach acid or non-acidic content refluxes frequently, it irritates the esophagus lining, leading to GERD.
- **Hiatal Hernia:** A stomach abnormality where a part of the stomach pushes up through the diaphragm muscle. It can increase the likelihood of acid reflux and subsequently GERD.

- **Overeating:** Consuming large meals can put pressure on the lower esophageal sphincter (LES), causing it to open and allow stomach acid to reflux.
- **Certain foods and drinks:** Certain items like fried food, fast food, pizza, chips, spicy foods, caffeine, and alcohol can trigger heartburn by irritating the esophagus or weakening the LES.
- **Being overweight:** Excessive body weight can exert pressure on the abdomen, pushing stomach contents into the esophagus.
- **Smoking:** Smoking can weaken the LES, making it easier for stomach acid to reflux.
- **Delayed stomach emptying:** Also known as gastroparesis, this condition can contribute to acid reflux as food and stomach acid can pool in the stomach, increasing the likelihood of reflux.

This list is not exhaustive, and there may be other factors that can contribute to acid reflux. If you experience frequent heartburn or any of the symptoms mentioned in the next section, it's essential to consult a doctor for proper diagnosis and treatment.

Symptoms of Acid Reflux

The most common symptom of acid reflux is heartburn, which may feel like a burning sensation in the chest. But acid reflux can also cause other symptoms, including:

- **Heartburn:** A common symptom of acid reflux, heartburn refers to a burning sensation in the chest, often after eating. This discomfort can intensify at night or when lying down.
- **Regurgitation:** This involves the backwash of stomach acid or undigested food reentering the mouth. It's an unpleasant sour taste that often occurs after meals.
- **Bloating:** Acid reflux can cause a feeling of fullness or swelling in the stomach. This uncomfortable sensation can lead to discomfort and reduced appetite.
- **Bloody stools or vomiting:** In severe cases of acid reflux, individuals may notice blood in their stools or vomit. This is often a sign of damage to the esophagus.
- **Burping:** Frequent burping is another symptom of acid reflux. The stomach acid irritating the esophagus leads to air being swallowed and subsequently belched out.
- **Dysphagia:** This term refers to difficulty swallowing. In acid reflux sufferers, the constant irritation and inflammation can make swallowing foods and liquids challenging.
- **Chronic cough:** A persistent cough, especially one that gets worse after eating or lying down, could be a symptom of acid reflux. This happens due to aspiration of stomach contents.

If you experience any of these symptoms regularly, it's crucial to seek medical advice. Early diagnosis and treatment can help prevent further complications.

Medical Treatments for Acid Reflux

Depending on the severity of acid reflux, doctors may prescribe medications to help relieve symptoms and prevent further complications. Some common medical treatments for acid reflux include:

- **Proton Pump Inhibitors (PPIs):** These prescription-strength medications, such as esomeprazole (Nexium), lansoprazole (Prevacid), and omeprazole (Prilosec), reduce the production of stomach acid. They can heal the esophageal lining in most people with GERD.
- **Antacids:** Available as a liquid or a chewable tablet, antacids neutralize stomach acid quickly to relieve heartburn symptoms. They are usually taken after meals.
- **Foaming agents:** Medications like Gaviscon coat the stomach to prevent reflux. They work by creating a foam barrier that helps block the reflux of stomach acid.
- **H2 Blockers:** Drugs like Pepcid and Tagamet decrease acid production. They can provide relief for mild to moderate symptoms of acid reflux.

- **GERD Surgery:** For severe GERD or when medications cannot help, surgery might be an option. This is usually a minor and effective procedure.
- **Lifestyle changes:** Eating sparingly and slowly, avoiding certain foods, and not drinking carbonated beverages can help manage acid reflux. It's also advised to stay upright after eating.
- **Over-the-counter antacids:** For quick relief of mild symptoms, over-the-counter antacids can be used. They work by neutralizing stomach acid.
- **Prescription medication:** Certain prescription medications like Dexlansoprazole (Dexilant), Esomeprazole (Nexium), and Omeprazole (Prilosec) are used to treat acid reflux. They work by reducing the production of stomach acid.

While medical treatments can help manage acid reflux, they may also have potential side effects. It's essential to discuss all treatment options with a doctor and regularly monitor symptoms.

Natural Remedies for Acid Reflux

If you prefer to manage acid reflux through natural remedies, various options are available. These remedies may not work for everyone, but they can provide relief for some people without potential side effects.

- **Honey:** Honey may soothe the esophagus by increasing mucus production and promoting healing, which can be beneficial in treating acid reflux and any resultant esophageal damage.

- **Herbal remedies:** Certain herbs like German chamomile, lemon balm, and licorice have been suggested as potential remedies for heartburn.
- **Chewing non-mint gum:** Chewing gum can stimulate saliva production, which can help neutralize stomach acid and keep it out of the esophagus.
- **Baking soda or apple cider vinegar:** Both substances have been cited as potential natural remedies for heartburn. Baking soda can neutralize stomach acid, while apple cider vinegar might help balance stomach acid levels.
- **Ginger:** Incorporating ginger into the diet has been suggested as another method to help manage acid reflux symptoms. Ginger has anti-inflammatory properties and might aid in calming the stomach.

These natural remedies may help manage acid reflux, but it's essential to consult with a doctor before trying them. Some herbs and ingredients may interact with medications or have adverse effects on certain health conditions.

Lifestyle Changes to Manage Acid Reflux

Along with medical treatments and natural remedies, making certain lifestyle changes can also help manage acid reflux. These changes may include:

- **Reducing stress:** High stress levels often exacerbate acid reflux symptoms. Engaging in regular stress-reducing activities like yoga, meditation, or light exercise can help alleviate these symptoms and promote overall well-being.

- **Avoiding late-night meals:** Eating meals or snacks too close to bedtime can trigger acid reflux. By avoiding late-night eating, individuals can give their bodies ample time to digest food properly, reducing the likelihood of nighttime reflux.
- **Quitting smoking:** Smoking can weaken the lower esophageal sphincter, leading to increased acid reflux. Quitting smoking not only strengthens this muscle but also contributes to better overall health.
- **Limiting alcohol consumption:** Alcohol has the ability to relax the lower esophageal sphincter and increase acid production in the stomach, both factors that can cause acid reflux. Curtailing the consumption of alcohol can notably lessen these risks.
- **Elevating the head while sleeping:** Elevating the head while sleeping can prevent stomach acid from flowing back into the esophagus. This simple adjustment can make a significant difference in managing acid reflux symptoms, especially during the night.

By making these lifestyle changes, individuals can help reduce the frequency and severity of acid reflux episodes.

What Is the Acid Reflux Diet?

The Acid Reflux Diet is a tailored eating plan aimed at minimizing the occurrence of acid reflux. This diet focuses on eliminating foods that trigger unpleasant symptoms and incorporating those that are less likely to provoke acid production in the stomach. It's not just about the types of food consumed, but also eating habits.

Regular, controlled meals and maintaining an upright posture after eating are part of the regimen. The goal is to alleviate discomfort and promote digestive health by making informed dietary choices.

In the next section, we will discuss the recommended food choices for an acid reflux diet, as well as those to avoid.

Principle of Acid Reflux Diet

Here are the key principles of the Acid Reflux Diet, each accompanied by a brief description to provide a better understanding of their role in managing gastroesophageal reflux disease (GERD):

- **Maintain a healthy body weight:** Excess weight puts pressure on the stomach, exacerbating acid reflux symptoms. By maintaining a healthy body weight, individuals can reduce this pressure and consequently mitigate the occurrence of acid reflux. Regular exercise and a balanced diet are key components in managing one's weight.
- **Avoid trigger foods:** Certain foods are known to exacerbate acid reflux symptoms, including tomato-based sauces, citrus fruits, chocolate, peppermint, and carbonated beverages. By identifying and avoiding these trigger foods, individuals can significantly decrease their acid reflux episodes.
- **Early meal times:** The timing of meals can influence acid reflux symptoms. Eating early allows the stomach to empty before lying down, reducing the chances of nighttime reflux. Small studies have shown that this principle can be beneficial in managing acid reflux.
- **Limit high-fat foods:** Foods high in fat, such as fried foods, high-fat baked goods, cream, ice cream, high-fat cheeses, sausages, bacon, and potato chips, can trigger acid reflux. By limiting the intake of these foods, individuals can help control their acid reflux symptoms.
- **Balanced macronutrients and micronutrients:** A balanced diet, rich in proteins, carbs, fats, vitamins, and minerals, can support overall digestive health and prevent acid reflux. Following a nutrient-rich diet ensures that the

body has all the necessary components for optimal digestion and absorption, thereby reducing the likelihood of acid reflux.

If these principles seem familiar, it's because they're recommended as part of a balanced and healthy lifestyle. The difference for those with GERD is that adhering to these principles may mean the difference between feeling uncomfortable or finding relief.

In the next section, we'll dive into the benefits of the Acid Reflux Diet.

Benefits of the Acid Reflux Diet

Below are the key benefits of following the Acid Reflux Diet, each with a brief explanation to help understand how this diet can aid in managing and reducing the symptoms of gastroesophageal reflux disease (GERD):

Reduced Symptoms

An acid reflux diet, specifically designed to alleviate the distressing symptoms of this condition, can bring about a significant reduction in heartburn and indigestion. This particular diet works by systematically eliminating foods that are known to trigger acid reflux, thus providing substantial relief for those who grapple with this condition daily.

By strictly adhering to this diet, individuals can witness a marked reduction not just in the frequency of these symptoms, but also in their severity. This means fewer episodes of discomfort and pain, and when they do occur, they're less intense. The diet essentially acts as a form of dietary management, helping individuals regain control over their health and well-being.

The beauty of this diet is its direct impact on the quality of life of those suffering from acid reflux. With reduced symptoms, individuals can enjoy meals without the constant fear of triggering an episode. This newfound freedom can greatly enhance their overall dining experience, making meal times pleasurable rather than a source of anxiety.

Improved Digestive Health

One of the main benefits of an acid reflux diet is its ability to reduce inflammation and promote better digestive health. This kind of diet regulates the production of stomach acid, which can have a significant impact on managing symptoms of acid reflux.

When stomach acid is kept at appropriate levels, it can prevent digestive discomfort, such as indigestion, bloating, and gas. Additionally, an acid reflux diet can help promote the growth of beneficial gut bacteria, leading to better nutrient absorption and regularity.

This is because healthy gut bacteria can assist in breaking down food and synthesizing vitamins and minerals. By incorporating this type of diet into your lifestyle, it can lead to significant improvements in digestive health and overall well-being.

Better Sleep

Incorporating an acid reflux diet is not only beneficial for reducing uncomfortable and painful symptoms, but it can also lead to better sleep quality. When acid production in the stomach is reduced by avoiding trigger foods, it allows for optimal digestion throughout the night. This means that the body will not be using energy to digest heavy or fatty foods, which can induce discomfort and disrupt sleep.

Additionally, acid reflux can cause disruptive and even dangerous nighttime breathing conditions such as sleep apnea. Incorporating an acid reflux diet can soothe the throat and airways, reducing the risk of respiratory disturbances during sleep. A proper acid reflux diet can also improve overall health and well-being, leading to a more restful and rejuvenating sleep.

Weight Management

By following an acid reflux diet that promotes weight management, individuals can reduce the frequency and severity of their acid reflux symptoms. In addition, maintaining a healthy weight has numerous health benefits, including reducing the risk of chronic conditions such as diabetes, heart disease, and certain types of cancer. An acid reflux diet can also improve overall digestion and nutrition by encouraging individuals to consume a balanced diet rich in nutrients.

Overall, an acid reflux diet that focuses on weight management can have significant benefits for individuals experiencing acid reflux symptoms. By adopting healthy dietary habits and maintaining a healthy weight, individuals can reduce their symptoms and improve their overall health and well-being.

Lower Risk of Complications

One of the most significant advantages of adopting an acid reflux diet is the decrease in the risk of complications associated with the condition. The esophagus is an essential part of digestive health and functions to move food from the mouth to the stomach with the help of muscular contractions.

Studies have shown that frequent exposure to stomach acid due to acid reflux can lead to inflammation and damage to the cells lining the esophagus, leading to more severe conditions such as esophagitis and Barrett's esophagus. By following an acid reflux diet, individuals can modify their diet to reduce the acidity level and avoid trigger foods, decreasing the chances of further damage to the esophagus.

Less Dependence on Medication

By following an acid reflux diet, individuals can experience the benefit of reduced dependence on medication. This is particularly significant considering the potential adverse side effects associated with long-term use of acid reflux medication.

The diet aims to minimize the production of stomach acid, thereby preventing symptoms such as heartburn, chest pain, and difficulty swallowing. By avoiding trigger foods and incorporating healthy alternatives, such as low-acid fruits and vegetables, lean protein, and whole grains, individuals may experience a significant reduction in the frequency and severity of acid reflux symptoms.

Moreover, the acid reflux diet promotes an overall healthier lifestyle, improving gut health and reducing inflammation in the body. Ultimately, adopting an acid reflux diet represents a natural and effective approach to mitigating the symptoms of acid reflux, reducing the need for medication, and promoting a healthier, happier life.

Encourages Balanced Nutrition

One key benefit of an acid reflux diet is the promotion of balanced nutrition. By avoiding trigger foods that can exacerbate symptoms, such as fatty foods or caffeine, individuals are incentivized to seek out healthier alternatives that provide the necessary vitamins and minerals for their overall health.

A well-rounded diet that includes a variety of nutrient-dense foods, such as whole grains, fruits and vegetables, and lean proteins, can lead to better absorption of nutrients and a decreased risk of chronic diseases like heart disease and diabetes. Additionally, a balanced diet can improve gut health and lead to healthier bowel movements. By sticking to an acid reflux diet, individuals can improve their overall nutrition and maintain a healthier lifestyle for long-term wellness.

These benefits highlight how the Acid Reflux Diet can have a positive impact on those suffering from GERD, leading to better overall health and reduced discomfort.

Disadvantages of the Acid Reflux Diet

While the Acid Reflux Diet offers notable benefits in managing GERD symptoms and promoting healthier eating habits, it also comes with a few potential downsides that are worth considering. Here are some of the disadvantages:

Limited Food Choices

Adhering to the Acid Reflux Diet poses certain challenges due to its restrictive nature, particularly when eating out or socializing. The limited food choices can result in feelings of deprivation and frustration, making it difficult for individuals to maintain the diet in the long term.

Research shows that adherence to the diet is strongly influenced by social factors, such as peer pressure and social support, highlighting the importance of support systems in helping individuals stick to the diet.

Potential Nutrient Deficiencies

It is important to note that those following an acid reflux diet may be at risk for nutrient deficiencies if not properly managed. For example, dairy products are often eliminated from the diet, which can lead to calcium deficiency and subsequent problems with bone health.

Individuals on this diet must work with a healthcare professional to assess and manage their nutrient intake to ensure optimal health.

Requires Discipline and Commitment

The acid reflux diet's demanding regimen can be a significant downside for those who find sticking to it challenging. The need for continued focus and attention can be daunting, as errant food choices may lead to severe bouts of reflux. Furthermore, this diet's rigidity can be time-consuming, leaving individuals struggling to maintain the necessary discipline for prolonged periods.

May Cause Weight Fluctuations

The downside of following an acid reflux diet is that it may cause unhealthy weight fluctuations. Some people may lose weight due to limited food choices, while others may gain weight from consuming high-calorie alternatives, leading to an imbalance in the body and potential health risks.

Therefore, it is important to maintain a well-balanced diet and consult a healthcare professional for guidance on weight management while following an acid reflux diet.

Can Be Costly

The cost of following an acid reflux diet can be a significant disadvantage for many people. Despite the numerous health benefits, fresh, organic produce and lean proteins tend to be more expensive than processed foods. This can pose a significant barrier for those on a tight budget and may limit the accessibility of a healthier diet for many individuals.

Despite these disadvantages, the benefits of the Acid Reflux Diet often outweigh the drawbacks. It promotes healthier eating habits, reduces inflammation, and improves digestive health. With careful planning and consideration, the disadvantages can be effectively managed, making the diet a viable option for managing GERD symptoms.

How to Get Started with the Acid Reflux Diet

If you're one of the millions suffering from acid reflux, it's time to take control. You can manage your symptoms and improve your quality of life by making dietary changes. Here is a simple 5-step plan to get you started on the acid reflux diet.

Step 1: Understand Your Condition

Before you embark on any dietary changes, it's critical to have a comprehensive understanding of the condition you're dealing with. Acid reflux, or Gastroesophageal Reflux Disease (GERD) as it's medically referred to, is a widespread digestive disorder that affects people globally. As mentioned, it is a condition characterized by the frequent backflow of stomach acid into the esophagus - the tube responsible for transporting food from your mouth to your stomach.

This abnormal reverse flow is commonly known as acid reflux. When it occurs, it can induce a burning sensation in the chest region, a symptom often referred to as heartburn. It's crucial to note that heartburn is not just an uncomfortable nuisance; it's a sign of an underlying issue that requires attention.

If acid reflux is left unchecked, the consistent backwash of harsh stomach acid can lead to irritation and potential damage to the lining of your esophagus. This damage can cause significant discomfort and may lead to more serious health complications over time.

Understanding the mechanics of acid reflux is essential because it provides a foundation for managing the condition effectively. It helps you grasp why certain foods exacerbate acid reflux and why others help to mitigate it. This knowledge ultimately guides your dietary choices, enabling you to select foods that will soothe rather than inflame your condition.

Moreover, knowing how acid reflux works can also help you understand the rationale behind other lifestyle recommendations for managing GERD, such as eating smaller meals, avoiding late-night meals, and elevating the head of your bed. These measures aim to minimize the amount of acid that comes into contact with your esophagus, thereby reducing the frequency and severity of heartburn.

In essence, a deep understanding of your condition is the first step towards effective management. It empowers you to make informed decisions that can significantly improve your quality of life.

Step 2: Identify Trigger Foods

Effective management of acid reflux hinges on the second crucial step: identifying foods that exacerbate your symptoms, often referred to as trigger foods. It's noteworthy to remember that these triggers can have varying effects among different individuals due to unique dietary habits, lifestyle choices, and genetic predispositions.

Therefore, gaining a thorough understanding of your body's specific reactions is of paramount importance. For instance, some people might experience an intensification of their symptoms after consuming certain types of food, such as spicy dishes or caffeinated beverages. Meanwhile, others might find that the same food items don't provoke any discomfort at all.

To identify your triggers, consider maintaining a detailed food diary. In this diary, record not only what you consume but also when you consume it, and most importantly, how it makes you feel afterwards. Be meticulous in your notes, capturing even seemingly insignificant details. You could note down the amount of food you eat, the time you eat, the combination of foods, and even your posture while eating.

Over time, as you review your entries, patterns may start to surface. These patterns can provide invaluable insights into which specific foods or eating habits trigger your acid reflux. Keep in mind that this process requires patience and careful observation. It's not about making quick changes but rather about gathering enough data to make informed decisions about your diet.

Remember, the ultimate goal isn't to drastically limit your food options but to establish a balanced, healthy eating plan tailored to your needs. By identifying your trigger foods, you can create a diet that not only contributes to your overall health but also helps keep your acid reflux symptoms under control. This way, you're not just avoiding discomfort, but also actively promoting better digestive health.

Step 3: Design Your Diet

After you've identified your trigger foods, the next constructive step involves designing a diet that not only caters to your taste preferences but also aids in managing your acid reflux symptoms. The primary goal here is to create a balanced diet comprising a variety of foods less likely to provoke your symptoms.

Lean proteins such as chicken or turkey are excellent choices because they're easy on the stomach and less likely to cause acid reflux. Whole grains like brown rice and oatmeal are also beneficial as they provide necessary fiber, which aids digestion and prevents constipation - a condition that can exacerbate acid reflux symptoms. Moreover, incorporating a diverse array of fresh fruits and vegetables into your diet ensures you receive essential vitamins and minerals, contributing to overall health and well-being.

Instead of adhering to the traditional pattern of having three large meals a day, consider adopting a more frequent, smaller meal pattern. This approach prevents your stomach from becoming overly full, a condition that can increase the likelihood of acid reflux. Smaller, more frequent meals allow for easier digestion and less pressure on the lower esophageal sphincter, the muscle that prevents stomach acids from flowing back into the esophagus. By preventing overeating, you're less likely to experience the discomfort associated with GERD.

Furthermore, it's advisable to avoid eating close to bedtime. Try to ensure your last meal or snack is consumed at least two to three hours before you plan to sleep. This practice allows ample time for digestion and reduces the likelihood of nighttime acid reflux, a scenario that can lead to disrupted sleep and negatively impact your overall well-being.

Remember, managing acid reflux isn't just about eliminating certain foods from your diet. It's about adopting healthier eating habits and lifestyle changes that contribute to better digestive health. By carefully designing your diet, you're taking an active role in controlling your acid reflux symptoms, improving your quality of life, and promoting your long-term health.

Step 4: Stay Hydrated

Proper hydration plays a pivotal role in maintaining overall health, and it's especially beneficial for individuals dealing with acid reflux. Consuming ample water throughout the day can help dilute stomach acids, thus reducing the risk of acid reflux. However, it's vital to find the right balance. Drinking large quantities of water all at once, particularly during meals, can cause your stomach to become overly full and potentially trigger reflux symptoms.

To sidestep this potential pitfall, it's recommended to sip small amounts of water consistently throughout the day. This method ensures that you remain well-hydrated while also minimizing the risk of exacerbating your acid reflux symptoms. Moreover, paying careful attention to your daily water intake can also aid digestion by helping break down food and aiding in the absorption of nutrients.

Another important factor to consider is the temperature of the water you consume. Some people may discover that extremely cold or hot drinks might trigger their symptoms, so experimenting with different temperatures could prove beneficial. It's essential to remember that managing acid reflux isn't about following a one-size-fits-all approach, but rather understanding your body's unique responses and adapting your habits accordingly.

By staying adequately hydrated in a manner that suits your individual needs, you can make a significant contribution to managing your acid reflux symptoms. Remember, every small step you take towards maintaining proper hydration counts towards achieving better digestive health. This practice not only helps manage your symptoms but also contributes to your overall well-being, making you feel healthier and more comfortable throughout the day.

Step 5: Monitor Your Progress

The final, yet crucial step in managing acid reflux involves diligent and consistent monitoring of your progress. As you implement adjustments to your diet and lifestyle, it's essential to keep a vigilant eye on how these changes are affecting your symptoms. Maintaining a detailed record of your daily food and drink intake, as well as noting any fluctuations in your acid reflux symptoms, can prove invaluable. This practice will help you identify what dietary choices and lifestyle habits work best for your body and where further modifications may be necessary.

Despite all your efforts, if you find yourself still grappling with discomfort, or if your symptoms take a turn for the worse, don't hesitate to seek professional help. A registered dietitian or healthcare provider can offer personalized guidance based on your specific circumstances. They possess the expertise to assist in refining your dietary plan, suggesting suitable alternatives, and providing support throughout your journey towards better digestive health.

Remember, managing acid reflux is a gradual process, and everyone's body responds differently to changes in diet and lifestyle. It's perfectly okay to go through periods of trial and error as you figure out the best approach for your unique needs. Your perseverance and commitment to understanding your body's responses can significantly contribute to improving your quality of life.

The key to successful management of acid reflux lies in patience, observation, and consistency. It's about learning from each episode, making informed decisions, and constantly fine-tuning your approach. Every small improvement is a step forward toward your goal, and every challenge faced is an opportunity for learning and growth. By staying committed to monitoring your progress, you're not just managing your acid reflux symptoms but also actively contributing to your overall health and well-being.

By following this 5-step plan, you can successfully navigate the acid reflux diet, improving your symptoms and overall health. It may take time and patience, but the results will be worth it.

Please note that while the acid reflux diet can help manage symptoms, it should not replace medical treatment. Always consult with a healthcare provider for a comprehensive treatment plan.

Foods to Eat

Now that you have a better understanding of how to get started with the acid reflux diet, let's take a closer look at the types of foods you should be incorporating into your meals.

- **Lean Proteins:** Choose lean protein options such as chicken, fish, beans, and lentils instead of fatty meats like bacon and beef.
- **Whole grains:** Opt for whole grain options like brown rice, whole wheat bread, and quinoa instead of processed grains.
- **Fruits and vegetables:** Enjoy a variety of fruits and vegetables, as they are rich in vitamins, minerals, and fiber. However, be sure to avoid trigger foods such as citrus fruits and tomatoes.
- **Healthy fats:** Incorporate healthy fats from sources such as avocados, olive oil, and nuts. These can help reduce inflammation in the body.

By including these types of foods in your diet, you can improve your digestive health and manage acid reflux symptoms. It's essential to also pay attention to portion sizes and avoid overeating, as this can put excess pressure on the stomach and increase the likelihood of acid reflux.

Foods to Avoid

On the flip side, here are some foods that you should try to avoid or limit as much as possible to manage your acid reflux symptoms:

- **High-fat foods:** Fried foods, fatty cuts of meat, processed snacks, and high-fat dairy products can all be triggers for acid reflux.
- **Spicy foods:** Peppers and spices can irritate the digestive system, leading to symptoms of acid reflux.
- **Citrus fruits:** Oranges, grapefruits, lemons, and other citrus fruits can increase stomach acid production and worsen acid reflux.
- **Tomatoes:** While tomatoes are a great source of vitamins and antioxidants, they are also acidic and can trigger acid reflux in some individuals.
- **Caffeine:** Coffee, tea, and other caffeinated drinks can relax the lower esophageal sphincter (LES), causing stomach acid to flow back into the esophagus.
- **Alcohol:** All types of alcohol can irritate the lining of the stomach and increase acid production. Avoid or limit your intake to manage acid reflux symptoms.

By avoiding these trigger foods and incorporating healthy, whole foods into your diet, you can effectively manage your acid reflux and improve your overall health.

In the next chapter, we will provide a meal plan with sample recipes to help you get started on the acid reflux diet. Remember, everyone's dietary needs and preferences are different, so feel free to make adjustments that work for you.

Sample Meal Plan

To give you an idea of what a day on the acid reflux diet might look like, here is a sample meal plan with some delicious and easy-to-prepare recipes.

Here's a 7-day sample meal plan for someone dealing with acid reflux:

Sunday

Breakfast: A bowl of oatmeal topped with sliced bananas and a drizzle of honey.

Lunch: Grilled chicken salad dressed lightly with olive oil and lemon juice.

Dinner: Baked salmon with a side of steamed broccoli and quinoa.

Monday

Breakfast: Scrambled eggs (made with just the egg whites) and whole grain toast.

Lunch: Turkey and spinach wrap on a whole wheat tortilla.

Dinner: Grilled fish with a side of sweet potatoes and steamed green beans.

Tuesday

Breakfast: Smoothie made with spinach, pineapple, and coconut water.

Lunch: Quinoa salad with cucumber, tomatoes, and feta cheese.

Dinner: Roasted chicken breast with a side of roasted carrots and brown rice.

Wednesday

Breakfast: Whole grain cereal with almond milk and blueberries.

Lunch: Tuna salad served on a bed of lettuce.

Dinner: Baked cod with a side of steamed asparagus and couscous.

Thursday

Breakfast: Greek yogurt topped with honey and sliced almonds.

Lunch: Chicken soup with lots of vegetables.

Dinner: Grilled shrimp skewers with a side of quinoa and sautéed spinach.

Friday

Breakfast: Avocado and egg white toast on whole grain bread.

Lunch: Lentil soup with a side of whole grain bread.

Dinner: Baked turkey with a side of mashed cauliflower and steamed Brussels sprouts.

Saturday

Breakfast: Smoothie made with banana, almond milk, and a scoop of protein powder.

Lunch: Grilled chicken Caesar salad (with light dressing).

Dinner: Grilled tofu with a side of brown rice and steamed broccoli.

For snacks throughout the day, they can have low-acid fruits like bananas melons, or almonds. They should also make sure to stay hydrated by drinking plenty of water.

Remember, it's always best to consult with a healthcare provider or a dietitian when making significant changes to the diet. This plan is just a guide and individual food reactions can vary.

Sample Recipes

Banana Oatmeal

Ingredients:

- 1 cup oats
- 2 cups water or almond milk
- 1 ripe banana
- 1 tbsp honey

Instructions:

1. In a medium-sized pot, bring the water or almond milk to a boil.

2. Reduce the heat to medium and stir in the oats.

3. Cook the oats, stirring occasionally, for about 10 minutes until the oats are your desired thickness.

4. While the oats are cooking, slice the banana into small pieces.

5. Once the oatmeal is done, remove it from the heat and stir in the sliced banana.

6. Sweeten your banana oatmeal with a drizzle of honey, and serve it warm.

Grilled Chicken Salad

Ingredients:

- A pair of skinless, boneless chicken fillets
- Season with salt and pepper as per preference
- 1 tablespoon of oil from olives
- Approximately 6 cups of mixed salad leaves
- A cup of halved cherry tomatoes
- Half a cucumber, sliced
- Thinly sliced quarter of a red onion
- Salad dressing of your choice

Instructions:

1. Preheat your grill or grill pan over medium heat.

2. Season the chicken breasts on both sides with salt and pepper.

3. Lightly oil the grill or grill pan. Place the chicken on the grill and cook for 6-7 minutes on each side, until the chicken is cooked through and no longer pink in the middle.

4. Remove the chicken from the grill and let it rest for a few minutes. Then, slice the chicken into strips.

5. While the chicken is resting, prepare the salad. In a large bowl, combine the salad greens, cherry tomatoes, cucumber, and red onion.

6. Add the grilled chicken to the salad. Drizzle your favorite salad dressing over the top and toss to combine.

7. Serve the salad immediately, while the chicken is still warm.

Baked Salmon with Broccoli and Quinoa

Ingredients:

- 2 salmon fillets
- 1 tablespoon olive oil
- Salt and pepper to taste
- 1 head of broccoli, cut into florets
- 1 cup quinoa
- 2 cups water

Instructions:

1. Preheat your oven to 400°F (200°C).

2. Place the salmon fillets on a baking sheet. Drizzle with olive oil and season with salt and pepper. Bake for 12-15 minutes, until the salmon is cooked through.

3. While the salmon is baking, steam the broccoli until tender, about 5-7 minutes.

4. Rinse the quinoa under cold water until the water runs clear. Bring the quinoa and 2 cups of water to a boil in a medium saucepan. Reduce the heat to low, cover, and simmer until the quinoa is tender and the water has been absorbed for about 15 minutes.

5. Serve the baked salmon with the steamed broccoli and cooked quinoa.

Scrambled Egg Whites on Toast

Ingredients:

- 4 egg whites
- Salt and pepper to taste
- 1 teaspoon olive oil
- 2 slices whole grain bread

Instructions:

1. In a bowl, whisk the egg whites until foamy. Season with salt and pepper.

2. Heat the olive oil in a non-stick skillet over medium heat. Add the egg whites and cook, stirring constantly, until they are set but still soft, about 3-4 minutes.

3. While the eggs are cooking, toast the bread.

4. Serve the scrambled egg whites on the toast.

Turkey and Spinach Wrap

Ingredients:

- 1 spinach wrap or tortilla
- 2 slices of turkey
- Handful of fresh spinach leaves
- 1/4 red bell pepper, thinly sliced
- 2 tablespoons of cream cheese
- 1 tablespoon of feta cheese
- 1 tablespoon of chopped olives
- 1/2 teaspoon of dried oregano

Instructions:

1. In a bowl, combine the cream cheese, feta cheese, olives, and oregano. Mix until well combined.

2. Spread the cream cheese mixture evenly over the entire tortilla or wrap.

3. Layer the turkey slices on top of the cream cheese mixture.

4. Add the spinach leaves and red bell pepper slices.

5. Starting from the bottom edge, tightly roll up the tortilla or wrap.

6. Cut the wrap in half and serve.

Grilled Fish with Sweet Potatoes

Ingredients:

- 2 fish fillets (like salmon or halibut)
- Olive oil for brushing
- Salt and pepper to taste
- 2 medium sweet potatoes
- 1 tablespoon butter
- Fresh herbs for garnish (optional)

Instructions:

1. Preheat your grill to medium-high heat.

2. Brush both sides of the fish fillets with olive oil and season with salt and pepper. Set aside.

3. Wash the sweet potatoes and poke a few holes in them with a fork. Microwave them for about 5 minutes until they are just starting to soften.

4. Cut the sweet potatoes in half lengthwise and brush the cut sides with a bit of olive oil.

5. Place the fish and sweet potatoes (cut side down) on the grill. Cook the fish for about 4-5 minutes per side, or until the fish is opaque and flakes easily with a fork. Cook the sweet potatoes for about 15 minutes, or until they are tender and have nice grill marks.

6. Remove the fish and sweet potatoes from the grill. Add a bit of butter to the sweet potatoes while they're still hot.

7. Serve the grilled fish with the grilled sweet potatoes, garnished with fresh herbs if desired.

Spinach Pineapple Smoothie

Ingredients:

- 1/2 cup unsweetened almond milk
- 1/3 cup nonfat plain Greek yogurt
- 1 cup baby spinach
- 1 cup frozen banana slices (about 1 medium banana)
- 1 cup freshly cut pineapple
- Optional: 1 tablespoon protein powder or flax seeds for added nutrition

Instructions:

1. Place almond milk, Greek yogurt, spinach, slices of banana, and pineapple at the base of a blender.

2. If using, add the protein powder or flax seeds.

3. Blend until smooth. Taste and adjust the sweetness if needed.

Quinoa Salad

Ingredients:

- 2 cups cooked quinoa (cold)
- 2 cups fresh spinach leaves, chopped
- 1 cup chickpeas, rinsed and drained
- 1 red bell pepper, diced
- 1 cucumber, chopped
- A handful of cherry or grape tomatoes, halved
- A bunch of fresh parsley, chopped
- Juice of 1 lemon
- Olive oil, salt, and pepper to taste
- Optional: Feta cheese for topping

Instructions:

1. In a large bowl, combine the cooked quinoa, chopped spinach, chickpeas, diced red bell pepper, chopped cucumber, halved tomatoes, and chopped parsley.

2. Drizzle the salad with the juice of 1 lemon and a bit of olive oil. Season with salt and pepper to taste. Toss everything together until well mixed.

3. If using, top the salad with some crumbled feta cheese.

4. Serve the quinoa salad cold. It can be stored in the fridge for up to a few days, making it perfect for meal prep.

Roasted Chicken with Carrots and Rice

Ingredients:

- 1 whole fresh chicken, approximately 4 lb
- 3-4 whole carrots, shredded or chopped
- 1 onion, chopped
- 2-3 tablespoons of honey
- 1 tablespoon Dijon mustard
- Chili powder to taste
- Salt and pepper to taste
- 1 cup of brown rice
- Olive oil

Instructions:

1. Preheat your oven to 400 degrees F (200 degrees C).

2. In a compact bowl, blend the honey, dijon mustard, and chili powder, along with salt and pepper.

3. Rub the chicken with the honey mixture, making sure to cover all areas.

4. Place the chicken in a roasting pan. Add the chopped carrots and onion around the chicken.

5. Drizzle some olive oil over the vegetables and season them with salt and pepper.

6. Place the roasting pan in the preheated oven and roast for about 1 hour and 15 minutes, or until the chicken is cooked through.

7. While the chicken is roasting, cook the brown rice according to the package instructions.

8. Once everything is done, serve the roasted chicken with the carrots and brown rice.

Whole Grain Cereal with Almond Milk

Ingredients:

- 1 cup of your favorite whole-grain cereal
- 1 to 1 1/2 cups of almond milk (unsweetened or sweetened, as per your preference)
- Optional toppings: fresh fruits (like berries or banana slices), nuts, seeds, or a drizzle of honey

Instructions:

1. Start by pouring your selected whole-grain cereal into a bowl.

2. Pour the almond milk over the cereal. You can adjust the amount of milk to suit your preference.

3. Stir the cereal and milk together to combine.

4. If you wish, add your choice of toppings - fresh fruits, nuts, seeds, or a touch of honey can all add extra flavor and nutritional benefits.

5. Enjoy immediately while the cereal is still crunchy!

Tuna Salad

Ingredients:

- 2 cans of tuna in water (5 ounces each)
- 1/4 cup of mayonnaise
- 1 stalk of celery, finely chopped
- 1/4 of red onion, finely chopped
- 1 tablespoon of lemon juice
- Salt and pepper to taste

Instructions:

1. Drain the tuna well.
2. Mix the drained tuna, mayonnaise, celery, and red onion in a medium bowl until well combined.
3. Add the lemon juice, then season with salt and pepper to taste.
4. Mix again until everything is evenly distributed.
5. You can serve it immediately, or cover and refrigerate to let the flavors meld together for an hour or two before serving.
6. Enjoy this tuna salad on its own, on a bed of greens, or in a sandwich or wrap. It's a versatile, protein-packed meal option.

Baked Cod with Asparagus

Ingredients:

- 4 cod fillets
- 1 bunch of asparagus, trimmed
- 2 tablespoons of olive oil
- Salt and pepper to taste
- 2 cloves of garlic, minced
- 1 lemon, zested and juiced
- 2 tablespoons of fresh parsley, chopped

Instructions:

1. Preheat your oven to 400 degrees F (200 degrees C).
2. Arrange the asparagus in a single layer on a baking sheet. Drizzle with 1 tablespoon of olive oil, and sprinkle with salt and pepper. Toss to coat and then spread them out again.
3. Lay the cod fillets on top of the asparagus. Drizzle with the remaining olive oil and season with salt and pepper.
4. Sprinkle the minced garlic evenly over the cod and asparagus. Then sprinkle with lemon zest.
5. Bake in the preheated oven for about 12-15 minutes, or until the cod is opaque and flakes easily with a fork.
6. Drizzle the baked cod and asparagus with fresh lemon juice and garnish with chopped parsley before serving.

Greek Yogurt with Honey and Almonds

Ingredients:

- 1 cup of Greek yogurt
- 2 tablespoons of honey
- 1/4 cup of sliced almonds

Instructions:

1. Scoop the Greek yogurt into a bowl.
2. Drizzle the honey over the Greek yogurt.
3. Sprinkle the sliced almonds on top.

Chicken Vegetable Soup

Ingredients:

- 2 tablespoons of olive oil
- 1 onion, chopped
- 2 carrots, peeled and sliced
- 2 stalks of celery, sliced
- 2 cloves of garlic, minced
- 1 pound of chicken breast, cubed
- 1 teaspoon of salt
- 1/2 teaspoon of black pepper
- 6 cups of chicken broth
- 1 bay leaf
- 1 cup of green beans, chopped
- 1 cup of corn kernels
- 1 cup of peas

Instructions:

1. Heat the olive oil in a large pot over medium heat. Add the onion, carrots, and celery and cook until the vegetables start to soften about 5 minutes.
2. Add the garlic, cubed chicken, salt, and pepper. Cook until the chicken is no longer pink on the outside.
3. Add the chicken broth and bay leaf. Bring the soup to a boil.
4. Once boiling, reduce the heat to low and let it simmer for about 20 minutes.

5. Add the green beans, corn, and peas. Let the soup simmer for another 10 minutes, or until the vegetables are tender.
6. Remove the bay leaf before serving.

Grilled Shrimp Skewers

Ingredients:

- 1 pound of shrimp, peeled and deveined
- 1/4 cup of olive oil
- 1 teaspoon of lemon zest
- 1/4 cup of fresh lemon juice
- 3 tablespoons of honey
- 3 cloves of garlic, minced
- Salt and pepper to taste

Instructions:

1. In a large bowl, combine olive oil, lemon zest, lemon juice, honey, minced garlic, salt, and pepper.
2. Add the shrimp to the bowl and mix well to coat them with the marinade. Allow them to marinate for at least 15 minutes.
3. Preheat your grill to medium-high heat.
4. Thread the shrimp onto skewers.
5. Grill the skewers for 2-3 minutes on each side, until the shrimp turn pink.
6. Serve your grilled shrimp skewers immediately.

Please note: If you're using wooden skewers, make sure to soak them in water for at least 30 minutes before preventing them from burning.

Teriyaki Shrimp Sushi Bowl

Ingredients:

For the Teriyaki Sauce:

- 1/4 cup low-sodium soy sauce
- 2 tablespoons honey
- 1 tablespoon ginger, minced
- 1 clove garlic, minced
- 1 tablespoon cornstarch mixed with 1 tablespoon cold water (optional, for thickening)

For the Sushi Bowl:

- 1 cup sushi rice or any short-grain rice
- 2 cups water
- 1 pound shrimp, peeled and deveined
- 1 avocado, sliced
- 1 cucumber, thinly sliced
- 1 carrot, julienned
- 2 green onions, chopped
- Sesame seeds for garnish

Instructions:

1. In a small saucepan, combine the soy sauce, honey, ginger, and garlic. Bring to a simmer over medium heat. If you prefer a thicker sauce, stir in the cornstarch-water mixture and continue cooking until the sauce thickens. Set aside.

2. Rinse the rice under cold water until the water runs clear.
3. Add the rice and water to a saucepan and bring to a boil. Reduce heat to low, cover, and let it simmer for 20 minutes, or until the water is absorbed and the rice is tender. Let it cool slightly.
4. Heat a pan over medium heat. Add the shrimp and half of the teriyaki sauce, stirring to coat.
5. Cook for 2-3 minutes on each side, or until the shrimp are pink and cooked through.
6. Divide the cooked rice into four bowls. Top each bowl with equal portions of the cooked shrimp, avocado slices, cucumber slices, and carrots.
7. Drizzle the remaining teriyaki sauce over the top.
8. Sprinkle chopped green onions and sesame seeds over each bowl.
9. Serve immediately and enjoy your Teriyaki Shrimp Sushi Bowl.

Chicken and Mushroom Cheese Bake

Ingredients:

- Four chicken breasts, boneless and skinless
- Season with salt and pepper according to your preference
- 2 tablespoons of olive oil
- One diced onion
- Minced garlic, three cloves
- Sliced fresh mushrooms, amounting to 2 cups
- A cup of heavy cream
- Grated Parmesan cheese, one cup
- One cup of shredded mozzarella cheese
- Fresh parsley to garnish

Instructions:

1. Preheat your oven to 375°F (190°C) and lightly grease a baking dish.
2. Season both sides of the chicken breasts with salt and pepper.
3. In a large skillet, heat the olive oil over medium heat. Add the chicken breasts and cook for about 5-7 minutes on each side, until golden brown. Remove the chicken from the skillet and set it aside.
4. In the same skillet, add the diced onion, minced garlic, and sliced mushrooms. Sauté them until the onions are translucent and the mushrooms are tender.

5. Pour in the heavy cream, then stir in the Parmesan and half of the mozzarella cheese. Stir until the cheese is melted and the sauce is well combined.
6. Place the sautéed chicken breasts in the greased baking dish. Pour the mushroom and cheese mixture over the chicken.
7. Sprinkle the remaining mozzarella cheese over the top. Bake in the preheated oven for 25-30 minutes, or until the chicken is cooked through and the cheese is bubbly and golden.
8. Garnish with fresh parsley before serving. Your Chicken and Mushroom Cheese Bake is now ready to enjoy!

Maple BBQ Salmon

Ingredients:

For the Salmon:

- 4 salmon fillets
- Salt and pepper to taste

For the Maple BBQ Sauce:

- 1/2 cup maple syrup
- 1/4 cup BBQ sauce
- 2 tablespoons apple cider vinegar
- 2 cloves garlic, minced
- 1 teaspoon smoked paprika
- 1/2 teaspoon ground black pepper

Instructions:

1. In a small cooking pot, blend the maple syrup, barbeque sauce, apple cider vinegar, finely chopped garlic, smoked paprika, and ground black pepper.
2. Over medium heat, allow the mixture to reach a gentle simmer while stirring from time to time.
3. Let it cook for roughly 5 minutes or until the sauce has gained a bit of thickness. Once done, take it off the heat and keep it aside.
4. If you're using a grill, preheat it to medium-high heat. If you're using an oven, preheat it to 400°F (200°C).

5. Season both sides of the salmon fillets with salt and pepper.
6. Place the salmon fillets skin-side down on the preheated grill or in a baking dish if using an oven. Cook for about 4-5 minutes.
7. Brush the top of each salmon fillet with the Maple BBQ Sauce, then flip the fillets and cook for another 4-5 minutes, until the salmon is cooked through and flakes easily with a fork.
8. Serve the Maple BBQ Salmon hot, with extra sauce on the side. This dish pairs wonderfully with a fresh green salad or roasted vegetables.

Caribbean Fish Tacos

Ingredients:

For the Tacos:

- 4 white fish fillets (like mahi-mahi or cod)
- 8 small corn tortillas
- Salt and pepper to taste
- 1 tablespoon olive oil

For the Caribbean Salsa:

- 1 ripe mango, diced
- 1 red bell pepper, diced
- 1/2 red onion, finely chopped
- 1/2 cup chopped fresh cilantro
- Juice of 1 lime
- Salt to taste

Instructions:

1. Preheat your grill or stovetop grill pan over medium heat.
2. Season the fish fillets with salt and pepper on both sides, then drizzle with olive oil to prevent sticking to the grill.
3. Grill the fish for about 4-5 minutes on each side or until it's cooked through and easily flakes with a fork.
4. While the fish is cooking, prepare the Caribbean salsa.

5. In a mixing bowl, blend the chopped mango, crimson bell pepper, crimson onion, fresh coriander, and juice of lime. Mix thoroughly until well combined and add salt according to your preference.
6. Warm the corn tortillas on the grill for about 30 seconds on each side, then wrap them in a clean kitchen towel to keep them warm.
7. Once the fish is done, let it rest for a few minutes, then break it into bite-sized pieces.
8. Assemble your tacos by placing some grilled fish on each tortilla, then topping with a generous spoonful of the Caribbean salsa.
9. Serve immediately, with extra lime wedges on the side if desired.

Icy Mango Smoothie

Ingredients:

- 2 ripe mangoes, peeled and pitted
- 1 cup of ice cubes
- 1/2 cup of low-fat yogurt or almond milk (for a vegan option)
- 1/2 cup of orange juice
- 1 tablespoon of honey or agave syrup (optional)
- A pinch of salt

Instructions:

1. Cut the mango flesh into chunks.
2. In a blender, combine the mango chunks, ice cubes, yogurt/almond milk, orange juice, honey/agave syrup (if using), and a pinch of salt.
3. Blend until smooth and creamy. If the smoothie is too thick, add a bit more orange juice or water and blend again.
4. Taste and adjust the sweetness if necessary by adding more honey or agave syrup.
5. Pour the smoothie into glasses and serve immediately.

Note: Everyone's acid reflux triggers are different. If any ingredient doesn't suit you, feel free to substitute or eliminate it.

These sample recipes are just a small selection of the many healthy meal options available to help manage acid reflux through diet. By incorporating more whole grains, lean proteins, and fresh fruits and vegetables into your meals, you can reduce symptoms and improve overall health.

Experiment with different flavors and ingredients to find what works best for you. And remember, always consult with a medical professional if you have persistent or severe acid reflux symptoms. With a balanced diet and proper medical guidance, you can effectively manage acid reflux and live a healthier life.

Conclusion

Congratulations on reaching the end of this comprehensive guide on acid reflux and the acid reflux diet! You've taken a deep dive into understanding acid reflux, its impacts, and how to manage it through mindful eating. That's an impressive accomplishment, and you should be proud of your commitment to improving your health.

Acid reflux is more than just occasional heartburn or discomfort—it's a persistent issue that can significantly affect your daily life. But now, armed with knowledge and determination, you're equipped to combat its symptoms and reduce its impact.

Remember, you're not alone on this journey. Acid reflux affects millions globally, and like you, they are seeking ways to alleviate their symptoms. Every small change you make in your diet and lifestyle can lead to significant improvements in your comfort and well-being.

The acid reflux diet is not a one-size-fits-all solution. It's essential to remember that everyone's body responds differently to different foods. Keep a close eye on your body's reactions and maintain a food diary to identify your unique triggers.

Changing dietary habits is a gradual process, and consistency is crucial. If you don't see immediate results, don't lose heart. Keep experimenting, keep persevering, and most importantly, keep believing in the power of dietary changes to improve your health.

As we conclude, let's recap some key points. Certain foods can trigger acid reflux symptoms while others can help alleviate them. Eating smaller meals, avoiding late-night snacking, and maintaining a healthy weight can significantly reduce the frequency and severity of acid reflux episodes.

It's empowering to realize how much control we can exert over our health simply by making mindful dietary choices. By adjusting what, when, and how much we eat, we can greatly influence our body's functioning and overall comfort.

Remember to be patient with yourself as you embark on this journey of managing your acid reflux through diet. Change takes time and persistence, but each step you take brings you closer to a healthier, more comfortable life.

You've taken the time to educate yourself, to understand the relationship between diet and acid reflux. That's commendable. So, here's to you, to your health, and to your commitment to taking control of your well-being.

Thank you for being proactive in your health journey. Every step you take is a step towards improved health and a better quality of life. Keep going, keep learning, and keep striving for a healthier you.

FAQs

What is acid reflux?

Acid reflux, also known as gastroesophageal reflux disease (GERD), is a condition where stomach acid frequently flows back into the esophagus. This backwash (acid reflux) can irritate the lining of the esophagus, causing heartburn and other symptoms.

What causes acid reflux?

Several factors can lead to the development of acid reflux. These include being overweight, being pregnant, the habit of smoking, the use of specific medications, as well as the consumption of certain types of food and beverages. Foods and drinks that can trigger acid reflux include those that are high in fat or fried, tomato-based sauces, alcoholic beverages, chocolate, mint, garlic, onions, and products containing caffeine.

What are the symptoms of acid reflux?

Usual signs of acid reflux include a fiery feeling in the chest known as heartburn, a reverse flow of food or sour liquid, difficulties when swallowing, constant cough, wheezing, and unease in the chest area, especially noticeable when lying down during the night.

How is acid reflux diagnosed?

Doctors usually diagnose acid reflux based on symptoms. However, in some cases, certain tests such as an endoscopy, ambulatory acid probe tests, or an esophageal motility test may be required.

What is an acid reflux diet?

An acid reflux diet involves consuming foods that are low in acid and fat, and high in fiber. It aims to reduce symptoms of acid reflux by avoiding foods that trigger heartburn and other symptoms.

Which foods should be avoided on an acid reflux diet?

People with acid reflux should avoid foods and drinks that trigger their symptoms. Common triggers include spicy foods, fatty foods, citrus fruits, tomato-based foods, chocolate, mint, garlic, onion, and caffeine.

Can lifestyle changes help manage acid reflux?

Yes, lifestyle changes can significantly help manage acid reflux. These include maintaining a healthy weight, avoiding food two to three hours before bedtime, elevating the head while sleeping, avoiding clothes that are tight around the waist, and quitting smoking.

References and Helpful Links

Stuart, A. (2008, July 9). What is acid reflux disease? WebMD. https://www.webmd.com/heartburn-gerd/what-is-acid-reflux-disease.

Schipani, D. (2021, December 1). What's the difference between acid reflux and GERD? | Everyday Health. EverydayHealth.com. https://www.everydayhealth.com/gerd/symptoms/whats-difference-between-acid-reflux-gerd/.

8 foods to avoid with Acid Reflux and follow healthy lifestyle. (2021, March 9). https://www.pacehospital.com/8-foods-to-avoid-with-acid-reflux-and-follow-healthy-lifestyle.

Heartburn, acid reflux, or GERD: What's the difference? | Pfizer. (n.d.). https://www.pfizer.com/news/articles/heartburn_acid_reflux_or_gerd_what_s_the_difference.

Seymour, K. (2023, October 31). What Is Acid Reflux? Symptoms, Causes And Treatments. Forbes Health. https://www.forbes.com/health/conditions/acid-reflux/.

8 Home Remedies To Relieve HeartburnHome remedies for Heartburn: 8 Ways to get rid of acid reflux. (n.d.). https://www.houstonmethodist.org/blog/articles/2021/dec/home-remedies-for-heartburn-10-ways-to-get-rid-of-acid-reflux/.

Professional, C. C. M. (n.d.). Acid Reflux & GERD. Cleveland Clinic. https://my.clevelandclinic.org/health/diseases/17019-acid-reflux-gerd.

www.ingramcontent.com/pod-product-compliance
Lightning Source LLC
LaVergne TN
LVHW012034060526
838201LV00061B/4600